# Having a
# Baby

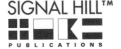

SIGNAL HILL™

PUBLICATIONS

Copyright © 1997
Signal Hill Publications
An imprint of New Readers Press
U.S. Publishing Division of Laubach Literacy International
Box 131, Syracuse, New York 13210-0131

Printed in the United States of America

Information graphics by Mark Kogut
Illustrations by Linda Alden
Cover photo: THE STOCK MARKET/Howard Sochurek
            1996
Cover design: Kimbrly Koennecke

9 8 7 6 5 4 3 2 1

Library of Congress Cataloging-in-Publication Data

Having a baby.
p. cm. — (For your information)
ISBN 1-56853-032-3 (pbk.)
1. Pregnancy. 2. Childbirth. I. Series: FYI (Syracuse, N.Y.)
RG525.B18      1997
618.2'4—dc21                        96-29521
                                        CIP

# Contents

# Preface

Information is power. Being informed means being able to make choices. When you can make choices, you have more power.

The information in this book can help you take control and make choices about your pregnancy and childbirth. The information will help you work with your doctor, nurse-midwife, or other care providers.

*Having a Baby* was developed with Sharron S. Humenick, Ph.D., RN, FACCE, Editor of the *Journal of Perinatal Education*. She has been a childbirth educator certified by ASPO/Lamaze since 1970 and has written articles and books on pregnancy and childbirth.

Thanks to the following people for their contribution to the content of *Having a Baby:* Dr. Richard Aubry, Director of Community Obstetrics, and Dr. Annette Pfannenstiel, Director of Pre/Perinatal Parenting Education Program, State University of New York Health Science Center, Syracuse, NY; Faith Terry, RNC, CE, Prepared Childbirth Consultants,

Liverpool, NY; Toni Cordell, New Reader Leadership Coordinator, Laubach Literacy; Michele Sedor, Health Coordinator, The Literacy Project, Greenfield, MA; Diana North and Donna Swain, The North Quabbin Adult Education Center, MA; and the Reverend Senitila McKinley, member, Laubach Literacy Action Steering Committee.

Thanks to Susan James and Jeanna Walsh for research and to Cynthia Moritz for writing.

## In this book

- *Prenatal care provider* refers to your doctor, nurse-midwife, family practice physician, or other medical provider you work with before the birth of your child.
- *Birthing care provider* refers to the care provider who attends the birth of your child. This is often the same person as your prenatal care provider.
- The word *partner* often refers to the father of the child. However, the partners of some mothers-to-be are women.
- If you do not have a partner, think about the person or people who are your most important supporters, or skip the sections about partners.

# Chapter 1

# Starting the Journey

Learning you're pregnant can be a happy time. But it's also a scary time. Having a baby will change your life forever.

With your first baby, you may have extra concerns, such as:

- Will I be a good parent?
- Will I have enough money to take care of a baby?
- Will I be able to cope with all the changes?
- How will my partner cope?

It's normal to worry. But take time to enjoy being pregnant too. Feel the new life move and grow inside you. Having a baby is a natural process. Your body is wise about the changes.

You're probably looking forward to becoming a parent months from now. But guess what? Everything you do from now on will affect your baby.

---

The moment you find out you're pregnant, you become a parent. You must start making decisions for both you and your baby.

---

Your doctor or nurse-midwife is there to help you through your pregnancy. Other women who have been pregnant can also give you helpful advice and share their experiences.

## Making Sure

If you are pregnant, it's best to know right away. That way you can start taking care of yourself and your baby.

Many women do a test at home. You can buy a home pregnancy test kit in any drugstore. Home pregnancy tests are usually right. But if a home test says you're pregnant, you should also get a pregnancy test at a clinic or health care office. That way, you can be sure.

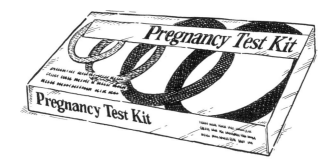

You may try a home test if you have physical signs of being pregnant. These include missed periods and swollen breasts. What if you have the signs, but the home test says you're not pregnant? In that case, you still might want to get a test at a clinic or health care office.

## Due Date

If you are pregnant, you will want to know the baby's expected due date.

Very few babies are born right on the due date. But the baby will be born within a couple of weeks before or after that date.

The average length of a pregnancy is 280 days. That's 40 weeks.

To figure out the due date, try to remember the date your last period started. (Many women

write that date down each month.) Then count
back three months and add seven days. This
chart shows the baby is due July 11.

| January | | July | ③ | 4 + 7 = 11 |
|---|---|---|---|---|
| February | | August | ② | |
| March | | September | ① | |
| April | | October | | 4 |
| May | | November | | |
| June | | December | | |

Maybe you don't know when your last
period started. Your care provider can measure
the size of the baby to figure out the due date.

## Breaking Bad Habits

Once you are sure you're pregnant, you
should see a doctor, nurse-midwife, or other
prenatal care provider. Chapter 2 gives advice on
finding a care provider. It may be a few weeks
before your appointment. But you must start
taking care of yourself and your baby right away.

First, make sure you're not putting anything
in your body that could harm your baby. Your
baby shares everything you put in your body.

☞ Drinking alcohol or taking drugs when you're pregnant can harm your unborn baby.

## Alcohol

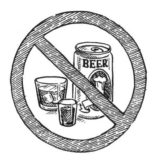

If you drink alcohol while you're pregnant, your baby could

- be mentally retarded
- be very small
- be weak and sickly
- become an addict
- have fetal alcohol syndrome (FAS). Children with FAS are often retarded and have other health problems.

## Drugs

If you use drugs while you're pregnant

- you may have a miscarriage

- you may bleed a lot during the birth
- you may have the baby too soon
- your baby may be very small and sickly
- your baby may have to go through drug withdrawal when it's born

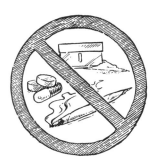

If you have ever injected street drugs, you may be at high risk for HIV (the virus that causes AIDS). You may pass it to your baby.

To get help to quit, call your local alcohol and drug abuse hot line. Or call the National Clearinghouse for Alcohol and Drug Information at (800) 729-6686 or the National Drug Treatment and Referral Line at (800) 662-HELP (English) or (800) 66-AYUDA (Spanish).

Even drugs you get from your doctor can be bad for your unborn child. Before you get a prescription, mention that you're pregnant. That may change the treatment. If you were taking medication when you found out you were pregnant, ask your doctor if you should stop.

Also be careful of taking nonprescription drugs. Before you take even an aspirin, ask your doctor or nurse-midwife if it's OK.

Be sure to tell any care provider that you are pregnant. Providers may make different decisions if they know.

Pregnant women should not have X rays unless it's vital. This includes dental X rays.

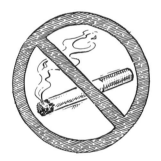

Smoking is bad for your unborn baby too. Each cigarette cuts down on the amount of oxygen and food carried to the baby. If you smoke when you're pregnant, the baby may

- be very small
- be stillborn (born dead)
- be born too soon

Seek help to quit. Call your local health clinic, or call the American Cancer Society at (800) 227-2345.

# Chapter 2

# Getting the Care You Need

## Your Prenatal Care Providers

You need to decide now who your prenatal health care providers will be. (*Prenatal* means *before birth*.) This means the doctors or nurse-midwives who will care for you during your pregnancy and may be with you at the birth.

Even if you don't have total freedom to choose a care provider, you may have some choice. Think about what things are important to you. That can help you decide what kind of care providers you would like.

## What kind of provider is right for you?

Do you believe that

- you should make most of the decisions, since it's your body and your baby?
- the care provider should make the decisions?
- the two of you should work together?
- you would prefer a woman to take care of you? Or a man?

There are three types of providers of prenatal care. They are described here:

**Obstetrician.** This is a medical doctor who specializes in treating pregnant women. If you want the doctor to be in charge, then you probably want an obstetrician. They are more likely than nurse-midwives and family practice physicians to take charge.

If you have problems during your pregnancy, you should see an obstetrician. Obstetricians have special training to deal with high-risk pregnancies. Those are pregnancies where there are likely to be problems because of the mother's medical history.

**Family practice physician.** This is also a medical doctor. A family practice physician's special training is in caring for all members of families. A family practice physician could also care for your baby after it's born.

A family practice physician has training to handle any normal pregnancy. If problems develop, he or she may refer you to an obstetrician.

**Certified nurse-midwife.** Certified nurse-midwives are registered nurses. They have training in caring for pregnant women and assisting in childbirth.

Nurse-midwives are trained to handle normal pregnancies. But if there are problems, the midwife should call in an obstetrician or family practice physician.

Do you want more say in decisions about your pregnancy? You may choose a family practice physician or nurse-midwife. Is it important to you not to treat pregnancy as a medical condition? A nurse-midwife may be the best choice.

## How to find a prenatal care provider

Say you have a general idea of the kind of care provider you want. Where can you find that person? You can

- ask people who recently had babies
- call your local health clinic

- call your local health department
- call the county medical society (Look in the white pages of the phone book.)
- call a nearby hospital that delivers babies. Ask for names of its attending physicians or nurse-midwives.
- call ASPO/Lamaze at (800) 368-4404. Ask for names of doctors or nurse-midwives in your area. The ASPO/Lamaze philosophy of birth is on page 94 of this book.
- call the International Childbirth Education Association at (612) 854-8660. Ask for names of doctors or nurse-midwives in your area.
- call the La Leche League at (800) LA-LECHE
- ask another health care provider, such as your doctor, dentist, or pharmacist

You can ask for providers who speak your native language. Some clinics and hospitals also have translators.

Once you have a list of a few prenatal care providers, talk to each one. You can prepare questions to ask. See page 18 for some ideas.

Try not to feel shy or afraid of asking all your questions. Practice them with a friend or family member. Take someone with you for your first visit if you can.

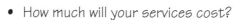

- How much will your services cost?
- How much time will you spend with me during each visit?
- Will you help me choose a healthy diet and level of exercise?
- How often will I have appointments?
- What kinds of tests do you do?
- Where will I deliver my baby? Can I choose?
- How much of a say will I have in decisions about the birth?
- What medical interventions do you use often during birth?

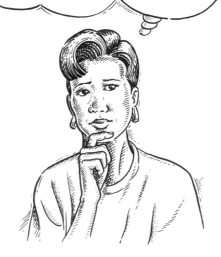

The answers to these questions are important. So is your feeling about the care provider. This is a person you will see several times. If you don't like the provider, move to someone else on the list.

If you don't have much say in choosing your care provider, try to have an open mind. Your care provider should give you the best care he or she can.

## The Birth Site

When you choose a care provider, most often you are choosing a birth site too. So while you are choosing a care provider, keep in mind where you want to give birth.

There are three basic choices for birth sites:

- hospital
- birth center
- home

### Hospitals

Most women in the U.S. give birth in hospitals. But in recent years, more women have chosen to have their babies in birth centers or at home.

Some hospitals use a labor room for women who are in labor. They then move the women to a delivery room for the birth. Many hospitals have created birthing rooms. These are sometimes called labor-delivery-and-recovery (LDR) rooms. These are rooms where a woman can labor *and* give birth. Many have wallpaper, curtains, and less of a "hospital" look. (This assumes you have a normal birth.)

At some hospitals, the new mother stays in the same room for her entire stay. She may be able to have her baby with her all the time.

---

Try to take a tour of the birthing section of the hospital where you will deliver. Get to know its layout so you know what to expect.

## Birth centers

A birth center is often separate from a hospital. It is usually run by nurse-midwives. Doctors are on call if they are needed.

Birth centers are more like home than hospitals are. A hospital may allow you to have your partner or another birthing coach in the room. But a birth center may let you have everyone you choose. Besides her partner, a woman can benefit from having an experienced woman present to support her. (Women who learn to help support mothers in labor are called doulas.)

Birth centers don't accept women whose pregnancies are high-risk.

## Home births

Some women choose to give birth at home. They want to be surrounded by family, friends, and their own things.

If your pregnancy is not high-risk and has been normal, a home birth is usually a safe choice. You should find a doctor or nurse-midwife who will attend a home birth. A nurse-midwife can tell you about planning a home birth.

Doctors and nurse-midwives are licensed by state law to attend births. In some places, unlicensed midwives help women with home births. They are not doctors or nurses. If you choose such a midwife, ask about her training, her qualifications, and her contact with a back-up doctor in case an emergency happens.

If you give birth at home, you must have a plan in case an emergency happens. You must have a vehicle and driver to get you to the nearest hospital quickly.

## Questions about birth sites

Here are some questions you might want to ask about your birth site:

- Can I have anyone I want present at the birth?
- Will the care I get respect my values, beliefs, and customs?
- Will I be able to move about freely and choose my position during labor and birth?
- Will the care providers help me use natural comfort measures before giving me medication or using medical procedures?
- Does this birth site know about community resources for new parents? Can it link me with these resources?
- Does the site encourage mothers to touch, hold, breast-feed, and care for their babies as much as possible?

## Dental Care

You need to see a dentist early in your pregnancy if you can. If your gums bleed when you brush your teeth, this is even more important. If you don't have a dentist, ask your care provider to help you find one.

# Chapter 3
# Medical Tests

Your prenatal care provider will probably want to do some medical tests during your pregnancy.

You can choose not to have many of the tests. It is your choice.

If you are healthy and between ages 17 and 35, your care provider may want to do only a few tests. But if you are older or your pregnancy is high-risk, she will probably want to do more. You decide how many tests you have. You may

- want every test to reassure yourself that the baby is OK
- want just the tests that your care provider can give you a good reason for having

## Standard Tests

Routine prenatal care includes asking for your medical history at your first visit. Your care provider will tell you about your pregnancy at each visit. He will also do standard tests and checks. Those are likely to include checking blood pressure, weight gain, the size of your uterus (womb), and urine blood sugar and protein. The tests are repeated at each visit. This makes sure the baby is growing well and your body is supporting the pregnancy.

Blood tests are commonly done during all pregnancies to check for

- **your blood group**

- **anemia** (lack of iron)

- **Rh factor.** If you have Rh factor in your blood, everything's OK. But if you lack Rh factor and the baby's father has it, your care provider will watch your pregnancy for problems.

- **rubella** (German measles). If a pregnant woman is infected, her baby can have serious health problems. If you haven't had rubella, stay away from anyone who has it while you're pregnant.

- **diabetes.** Some women develop this disease while they're pregnant.

- **hepatitis B.** This infection can cause serious health problems for you and your baby.

A Pap test will likely be done at your first visit. This tests for cancer of the cervix.

### Medical Tests for Pregnant Women

| | |
|---|---|
| **At each prenatal visit** | ■ blood pressure<br>■ weight gain<br>■ size of your womb<br>■ urine blood sugar and protein |
| **For all pregnant women** | ■ Rh factor<br>■ sickle-cell trait<br>■ rubella (German measles)<br>■ diabetes<br>■ hepatitis B |
| **Your care provider may advise** | ■ ultrasound<br>■ amniocentesis<br>■ AIDS screening<br>■ alpha-fetoprotein screening<br>■ chorionic villus sampling (CVS) |

## Tests You May Have

The following tests are not standard. You can choose *not* to have them in most cases.

**AIDS screening.** This is a blood test. You should have it if you might have HIV, the virus that causes AIDS. You are at high risk if

- you have had unprotected sex (sex without a condom) with someone who has the virus
- you are a drug user who has shared needles with anyone else

If you have HIV/AIDS, the earlier your care provider knows, the better. If you get early treatment, the chance of passing the HIV virus on to your baby can be reduced to about 10 percent. If you don't get treatment, the chance is 30 to 40 percent.

**Sickle cell screening.** People of African, Middle Eastern, Mediterranean, Caribbean, and Asian blood can carry the sickle-cell trait. If both parents carry it, the baby could have sickle cell anemia. People with this blood disease usually die at an early age.

**Ultrasound (sonogram, or "sono").** This test forms a picture of the baby and the placenta. It can be used to tell the baby's age and detect twins. It can also check on how the baby is doing.

**Alpha-fetoprotein (AFP) screening.** If this test is abnormal, the baby could have a birth defect. More testing should be done.

**Amniocentesis ("amnio").** This is most often done between the 15th and 18th weeks. A needle is inserted into the uterus. A small amount of fluid is withdrawn and tested.

Amnio can show whether a fetus has certain birth defects, including Down's syndrome.

Amnio is done most often when the mother is older than 35 or when the baby is at risk for a disease the test can find.

Amnio can be a risky test. Be sure you know the risks before you agree to have it.

**Chorionic villus sampling (CVS).** This test looks for many of the same things as amniocentesis. It can be done at the 10th or 11th week.

## Test or Not?

Consider the pros and cons of each test. Will it give you facts you want or need about the baby? You might want to know ahead of time if your baby is going to have a problem. Or you might prefer to deal with any problems after the baby is born. Page 28 lists some questions you might ask your care provider about any test.

☞ You have the final say on tests. Your doctor can give advice, but she needs your permission to do tests.

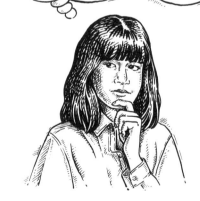

- What are you looking for with this test?

- Is this a standard test, or is there a special reason you feel I should have it?

- How is the test done? Where is it done?

- What are the risks of having this test?

- What is the cost, and who pays?

# Chapter 4

# Taking Care
# of Yourself

Everything you do while you're pregnant affects your baby. If you take good care of yourself now, your baby is more likely to be healthy.

## Eating Right

Write down everything you eat for two days. Then look at your list.

- Are there things on the list that you think will help your baby grow healthy, such as

fruit, vegetables, milk, and lean meats?
Circle them.

- Are there things on the list that you think
  won't help your baby grow healthy, such as
  soda, sugary snacks, potato chips, and
  drinks with caffeine? Underline them.

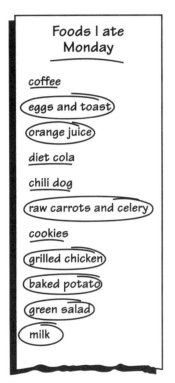
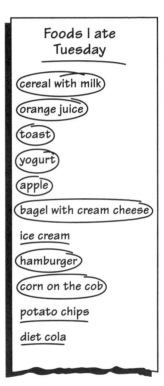

This exercise can show you what needs to
change in your diet while you're pregnant. Aim
to reduce the number of underlined items. Try
to increase the number of circled items.

Be sure to drink six to eight glasses of water or fruit juice a day. This helps your baby grow healthy.

- - - - - - - - - - - - - - - - - - - - - - - -
Your baby eats and drinks everything you do. - - - -

See pages 56 and 57 for information about programs that can help you pay for food.

## Calories for baby

For the baby to grow the way it should, most women should eat about an extra 300 calories each day. You may eat a little less than that early in the pregnancy and a little more during the last months.

Those calories should come from foods that are full of nutrients. Nutrients are the useful materials in food. It's especially important to get enough protein. Protein is used to build new tissue. You also need extra calcium, vitamins, minerals, and iron.

Your prenatal care provider will probably give you vitamins to take. These help your baby grow healthy.

You can talk with your prenatal care provider about what and how much it's best to eat. Try to stay away from soda, candy, chips, and other junk foods. They won't give you the nutrients you and your baby need. Soda also robs the body of calcium.

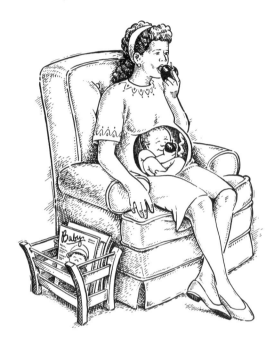

## Weight gain

Many women are concerned about how much weight they will gain while pregnant. They are worried that the weight will never come off again.

It's normal to worry about this. But you need to gain weight while you're pregnant. Otherwise, your baby won't get the calories and nutrition it needs to grow well.

# Food Guide Pyramid

## A guide to daily food choices

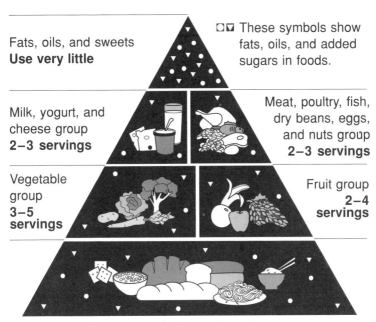

Fats, oils, and sweets
**Use very little**

☐🔻 These symbols show fats, oils, and added sugars in foods.

Milk, yogurt, and cheese group
**2–3 servings**

Meat, poultry, fish, dry beans, eggs, and nuts group
**2–3 servings**

Vegetable group
**3–5 servings**

Fruit group
**2–4 servings**

Bread, cereal, rice, and pasta group
**6–11 servings**

The Food Guide Pyramid can help you eat a balanced diet. The Pyramid lists the number of servings from each group you should eat each day. Pregnant women need about 300 extra calories a day. You should choose extra servings in the five main food groups to get these calories. This will help you get the extra protein, iron, and calcium you need. You don't need extra fats, oils, and sweets, though.

> ☞ Most women should plan on gaining between 20 and 30 pounds while they are pregnant.

You may gain little or no weight during the first three months. During the last six months, you should gain about a pound a week. But

- Overweight women should gain less.
- Underweight women should gain more.
- Teenagers, who may still be growing themselves, should gain more.
- Women carrying two or more babies should gain more.

If you have questions, ask your prenatal care provider what she thinks is right for you. You will lose most of the weight after the baby is born. Exercise and breast-feeding can help you lose any extra weight.

## Staying Fit

Most pregnant women can exercise safely. This is true even for women who didn't exercise before they became pregnant.

When you exercise during pregnancy, it can

- give you extra strength for labor, delivery, and recovery
- ease aches and pains in late pregnancy

- help you sleep better
- increase the circulation of blood through your body and to the baby

A few women shouldn't exercise while pregnant. They include some women who

- have high-risk pregnancies
- are very overweight
- are very underweight
- have another medical condition, such as heart disease or diabetes

---

Check with your prenatal care provider before starting or continuing to exercise.

---

If you already exercise, you can probably continue. But you will have to slow down as your pregnancy continues. And some sports should be dropped until after your baby is born.

Walking is a good way to stay fit. Many communities also have exercise classes for pregnant women. Ask your prenatal care provider if she knows of any.

When you exercise, you should follow some standard guidelines. These include warming up and cooling down, wearing the right clothes, and stopping if you feel pain.

Slow down in the last three months. Take it especially slowly in the ninth month. At this time, a little stretching and walking are enough.

## Coping with Your Worries

Every woman has fears and worries about her unborn baby. This can be even more true with a first baby. You might worry about being a good parent, coping with the pain of childbirth, or having a healthy baby.

Worries are natural, but don't let them take over your life. Don't let them stop you from taking care of yourself and the baby.

You can fight fears by

- getting as many facts as you can. For example, 98 percent of babies in the U.S. are born healthy. Knowing that might help you stop worrying about your baby's health.
- taking care of yourself—eating right, exercising, and seeing your prenatal care provider. Doing these things reduces the chance that anything will go wrong during the pregnancy or birth.

- learning to relax. Here are some ways to reduce stress: Get enough sleep. Talk out your worries with someone close. Take a walk or a warm bath. Breathe deeply and slowly. Play with a child or pet. Watch a funny movie. Take a nap.

## If You Get Sick

You may get some illness that has nothing to do with your pregnancy. It probably won't affect the baby. The illness may last longer than usual, though. That's because your immune system may not work as well in pregnancy. (Your immune system fights illness and disease.)

If you do get sick while you're pregnant

- drink a lot of fluids. If you are vomiting or have diarrhea, you can get dehydrated easily. Try to find some liquid you can keep down.

- eat if you can. Going without food for a day or two won't harm the baby, as long as you get enough fluids. But you may get better more quickly if you eat. Be sure to keep taking your pregnancy vitamins if you can keep them down.

- rest a lot.

- reduce a fever naturally. Take cool showers or baths, drink something cool, and wear light clothing. If your fever reaches 102 degrees, call your care provider.
- call your care provider if you have any illness that you're not familiar with.

---

Remember, don't take any medicine without your care provider's approval, even aspirin.

---

If your prenatal care provider tells you it is important to take a certain medicine, do it. Don't delay because you're afraid it might hurt the baby. But ask questions if you are worried. Be careful to take the correct dose.

# Chapter 5
# Big Changes

Having a baby will change your life in almost every way. It will affect

- your feelings about yourself
- your relationship with your husband or partner, if you have one
- your relationships with any other children you have
- your relationships with relatives and friends
- your work

## You and Your Partner

You may be nervous about how your partner will adjust to becoming a parent. He is probably nervous too.

While you're pregnant, most of the attention will be focused on you and the baby. Partners often feel left out during the pregnancy, and even after the baby is born. You can help your partner feel part of the pregnancy by

- asking him to come to your prenatal visits with you.
- taking childbirth classes together. Your partner will learn how to help you during labor and childbirth.
- telling him how you feel about the baby and what being pregnant is like.
- helping him make contact with the baby by feeling your belly and talking to the baby.
- shopping together for baby equipment and clothes.
- talking to him about your fears and worries. He may fear that something bad will happen to you or the baby during the birth. Or he may worry about how you and he will support a new baby.
- encouraging him to learn more about pregnancy and childbirth.

> If you take care of your relationship while you are pregnant, it will likely be stronger when the baby comes.

Pregnancy can be a difficult time for some couples. A few people become violent when their partner is pregnant. If you are being abused, seek help. Find out where your nearest safe house or women's shelter is. You may need to go there to protect yourself and your baby.

## Sex during Pregnancy

One of the things that will change during pregnancy is your sex life. But it's hard to know ahead of time exactly how it will change.

Some pregnant women have little or no desire for sex. They are focusing most of their thoughts on the baby. Some are afraid that having sex might hurt the baby. Other women want sex more while they're pregnant.

Any of these reactions is normal. Many women find that their desire for sex changes at different stages of pregnancy.

In most cases, it is safe to have sex all through your pregnancy. As your belly gets bigger, though, you may have to try different positions to be comfortable.

In a few cases, a pregnant woman may have to limit sex during pregnancy, such as:

- when there is any unexplained bleeding
- during the first three months if she has had miscarriages, or if there are any signs of a miscarriage
- during the last 8 to 12 weeks if she has had early labor before, or if there is any sign of early labor
- after her water has broken

## Other People in Your Life

Your relationship with some people will change when you become pregnant. You may grow closer to some people, especially women who have had babies. You will have more in common than you did before.

But it may be hard to stay close to some friends. It may hurt if other people aren't as excited about the baby as you want them to be. Most women change some friendships when they become pregnant. This is normal.

## Big Brothers and Sisters

If this is not your first baby, you'll need to prepare your older child or children. How an older child accepts the new baby will depend partly on how well he is prepared.

All children tend to get jealous when a new baby comes into their family. They may feel forgotten. They may feel that the new baby is more important or more loved. But you can do a lot to make the change easier for your older children.

Seek advice about preparing older children from your prenatal care provider or childbirth teacher. (Chapter 8, page 60, talks about childbirth education classes.) Preschool children and school-age children have different needs.

Here are some general tips for preparing children and making them feel included:

- Have them help you gather clothes and equipment for the new baby. Ask them to give ideas for the baby's name. Include them in some doctor visits.

- Allow your children to express their doubts and fears about the new family member. Be honest about your feelings, too.

- Talk about the new baby as "ours." Allow your children to touch your belly and feel the baby.

- Talk openly about what having a baby in the house will mean. Your other children will have to give up some of your time and attention. Be honest about this, but plan with them to have some special time together after the baby arrives.

- Be honest that a new baby is not much of a playmate. Explain that a new baby mostly eats, sleeps, cries, and fills diapers.

- When you come home with the new baby, be sure someone else carries the baby so you can greet the older children.

- Make any planned changes in beds or bedrooms weeks before the new baby comes.

- Ask your friends and family to pay special attention to the older children.

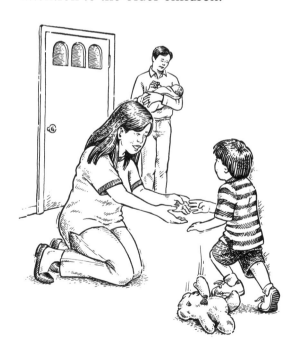

- Have little gifts ready to give your children when you get home and when visitors bring gifts for the new baby.
- Include your older children in caring for the new baby. Have them help by bringing you things.

Be prepared for your other children to act like babies again themselves. This will probably not last long. Do not feel bad if they do not seem to be happy about the new baby or to love it at first. It may take time for them to get used to it.

---

Remember, older children are likely to have some strong reactions to the new baby. Allow them to express themselves, and accept their feelings.

Keep the new baby safe. Do not leave preschool children alone with newborns. Show older children how to keep the baby safe.

Many childbirth teachers offer special classes to prepare children for the new baby. You can get information from your childbirth teacher or your prenatal care provider.

There are also many good books to help you prepare older children. Some books explain how the baby got inside you, how it grows, and how it's born. Other books deal more with older children's feelings about a new baby. Check your local library or bookstore for such books.

## Single Parenthood

Perhaps you are having a baby without a husband or other partner. Having a child may be harder for you than for women with partners. But many women have babies without partners and do fine.

It's helpful if you have friends or relatives to help you out. Someone close to you can

- attend childbirth classes with you and coach you during the birth
- run errands for you when you are feeling sick or when your energy is low
- provide support and listen to your worries and fears

There may be a club, program, or support group for single parents. Check with the health departments in your area.

---

Don't be shy about asking for help. Many people are happy to help out a new mother.

## Changes of Feelings

While your body is going through major changes, your feelings will, too. It's easy to predict what your body will be doing at each stage of pregnancy. But your feelings may change from day to day, or from hour to hour.

You may find yourself

- depressed for no reason you can think of
- worried about yourself and the baby
- very happy about the future
- breaking into tears over small things

If you find yourself having bad feelings (the blues) for a long time, mention it to your prenatal care provider. There may be a physical reason for your feelings. Your prenatal care provider may be able to help you or refer you to someone who can.

But if you're just moodier than usual, relax. It's normal to worry when you enter a whole new stage of life.

# Chapter 6

# Physical Changes

Here are some of the changes you can expect in your body as your baby grows. They are listed by trimesters. Trimesters are three-month periods. Pregnancy is often broken into trimesters.

## First Trimester (1st to 3rd Months)

The baby will grow to be three inches long and weigh about an ounce. Its major organs are forming. The heart is beating. It begins to move its hands, legs, and head. Testes form in boys, and ovaries form in girls. The external sex organs still look similar in both sexes.

You may not notice much change in your body during this time. You probably won't gain much weight. You might

- have a little bleeding or mucous discharge from the vagina. This is probably normal, but tell your care provider about any bleeding.
- feel sick to your stomach (or even vomit). You can get this "morning sickness" at any time of day.
- have swelling and soreness in your breasts.
- have pain in your lower back and legs.
- urinate more often than usual, and move your bowels less often.
- be more tired than usual.

## Second Trimester (4th to 6th Months)

The baby will grow to be about 14 inches and $1\frac{1}{2}$ pounds. Its eyelashes and nails will grow. It will be able to kick and suck its thumb.

You will start gaining weight, especially in the belly. You will probably have to start wearing maternity clothes. You may have trouble breathing sometimes. This is because the baby is taking up more space.

*1 month*

 *2 months*

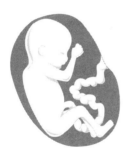 *3 months*

*4 months*

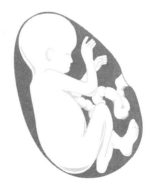 *5 months*

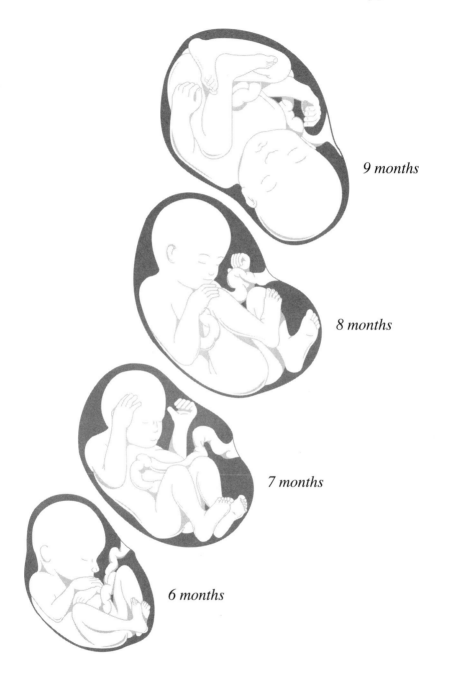

*9 months*

*8 months*

*7 months*

*6 months*

Pink or reddish lines may appear on your stomach. Your nipples may darken. They may leak a yellow fluid, called colostrum (early milk).

## Third Trimester (7th to 9th Months)

By the end of the seventh month, the baby's development will be almost complete. The baby's eyes will open. Its hair will grow longer.

In the eighth or ninth month, there are signs of getting ready for birth. The baby will probably turn so its head is down. You may feel your belly getting tight for a few seconds from time to time. These are Braxton-Hicks contractions. They don't mean you're in labor yet. The baby moves lower, getting ready for birth. You will probably be able to breathe more easily again.

Other things that will happen to your body in the eighth and ninth months include

- swelling of your ankles
- difficulty sleeping
- your navel getting pushed out

Knowing when you begin labor is covered in Chapter 10, page 76.

# Chapter 7

# Money and Work

## Paying for Pregnancy and Childbirth

There are three main ways that people pay for prenatal care and childbirth:

- health insurance
- Medicaid (a government health insurance program for people with low incomes)
- their own money

If you have health insurance, it may pay for much of your prenatal care and childbirth. Most health insurance plans don't cover everything, though.

> You should find out exactly which expenses your insurance covers. This will help you avoid costly surprises later on.

You can look at your policy to find out what is covered. But sometimes the policy is written in a confusing way. If you get health insurance through your job, talk to the human resources (personnel) department about what is covered. You can also call the insurance company.

Your insurance may cover just a certain percentage of each expense. You will have to pay for the rest yourself.

## If You Can't Afford Insurance

You may qualify for Medical Assistance, or Medicaid. Some people can get Medicaid if they have a certain income level or have other special needs. You can also get it if you get Public Assistance (PA) or Supplemental Security Income (SSI). Call or visit your local department of social services (welfare office) or health department to get details. Or go to any Medicaid office and ask for more information.

Medicaid covers a range of health care needs. You can get some prenatal care even before it is proved you can get Medicaid. Ask your local Medicaid office or your prenatal care provider for more details. There is also a national Prenatal Care Assistance Program to help you get the care you need. Call your department of social services for details.

## No insurance or Medicaid

If you can't afford health insurance, but your income is too high for Medicaid, what can you do? You have two choices:

- Find a part-pay clinic. They charge only what you can afford to pay. Call your department of health or social services.
- Talk to your care providers. See if you can work out a payment plan you can afford. It is very important to see a health care provider while you are pregnant.

## Making Ends Meet after the Birth

You should start to plan now for how to pay for the things your baby will need. The biggest expense for many people is childcare. Will you stay home to care for the baby? Ask yourself:

- Can I afford to stay home?
- Can I afford to work and pay for childcare?

- If I stay home with the baby, what will I give up? Where will money come from?

If you have a partner and you decide that one of you will stay home, ask yourselves:

- Which of us makes more money?
- Which of our jobs is more secure?
- Which of us could more easily find a new job when the baby is older?
- Can we adjust our work so that we can both work and have one person home most of the time?

## When There Isn't Enough Money

Maybe no matter what you decide about working, there still won't be enough money. Government programs may be able to help:

**Welfare.** Call your local social services department if you think you qualify for welfare.

**WIC** (Special Supplemental Food Program for Women, Infants and Children). WIC provides free food for pregnant or breast-feeding women and for children under age 5. It also offers help in getting health care services you need.

To find out if you can apply for help from WIC, call your local health or social services department.

**Food stamps.** These are coupons that can be used like money to help buy food. Call your department of social services to find out if you can get food stamps.

**Aid to Families with Dependent Children (AFDC).** This program gives money to families with children that cannot fully support themselves for certain reasons. Call your department of social services to find out how you can apply.

## Working while You're Pregnant

Pregnancy is not an illness. But some things are harder to do while you're pregnant. Your chance of giving birth too early increases late in your pregnancy if your job requires you to

- stand on your feet for long periods of time
- lift heavy objects

Does your job involve either of these things? If so, can you change your duties or how you work? Could you work just as well sitting as standing? Could someone else lift those boxes?

Your employer may have a written policy about pregnancy. Talk to your boss or the human resources department where you work.

You can ease stress on the job by

- wearing maternity support hose if your feet swell.

- keeping one foot on a low stool with your knee bent while you stand. This takes some of the pressure off your back.

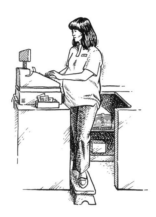

- keeping your feet elevated on a stool or carton while you sit.
- staying out of smoke-filled areas.
- taking frequent breaks.
- resting a lot when you're not working.

## If You Have to Stop Working

If you have problems in your pregnancy, you may have to stop working well before the baby is born. You may have to go on bed rest. That means staying in a lying position.

You may have to stop working if your job includes a lot of physical or mental stress.

If you have to stop working early, you may be able to get disability benefits. Talk to your boss or the human resources department where you work. Call the state department of labor office in your area to find out more about benefits.

## Your Maternity Leave

You will need to take some time off from work when the baby is born. Even if you want to return to work as soon as possible, your body needs time to recover from the birth.

If you can afford it, you might want to take a few months off. The Federal Family Leave Act guarantees workers 12 weeks of (unpaid) leave after the birth of a child if

- the company has at least 50 employees
- you have held your job for at least a year
- you have worked at least 25 hours a week

All parents (mothers *and* fathers) are entitled to this leave. Your jobs must be waiting for you when you return. However, your employer doesn't have to pay you during parental leave.

You may want to take more than 12 weeks off. If so, you and your employer will have to agree on the amount of time.

# Chapter 8

# Getting Ready

## Childbirth Classes

Taking a childbirth education class is especially helpful before the birth of your first child. A good class can

- reduce your fear of labor by giving you some idea of what to expect
- show you methods for relaxing during labor
- teach you skills that can help labor go faster and more comfortably

- teach you about the decisions you will have to make, such as whether or not to request pain medication
- tell you the basics of baby care
- help your partner get involved

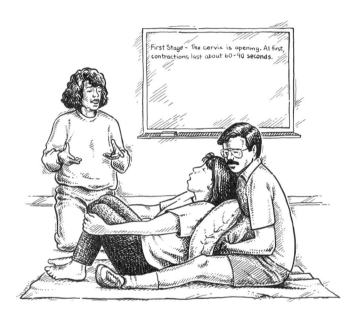

First Stage - The cervix is opening. At first, contractions last about 60-90 seconds.

The person who attends classes with you and learns how to help you during the birth is often called your coach.

You can find out about childbirth classes from several sources. They include

- your prenatal care provider
- the hospital or birthing center where you will deliver

• groups that have an interest in babies and childbirth, such as the La Leche League: (800) LA-LECHE or ASPO/Lamaze: (800) 368-4404

## Choosing a class

You can ask your prenatal care provider which class she recommends. Or talk to women you know who have recently had babies.

Keep the following things in mind:

**Class size.** Childbirth classes work best if they're small.

**Teaching methods.** Does the teacher use films of childbirth? Will you get a chance to talk to parents who have recently delivered? Is practice time provided during class?

**Certification.** Has the teacher passed a test for childbirth educators?

Try to find a teacher whose viewpoint you are comfortable with. Even if you can't find the ideal class, it's better to take a childbirth class than not. It will help you focus on the birth and the decisions you need to make.

## Making a Birth Plan

You don't know exactly what your baby's birth will be like. No one knows ahead of time how a labor will go. But you probably have some idea of what you would prefer. You can write what you prefer in a birth plan.

Some of the things you can say in a birth plan are included in the chart on page 64.

You should make your birth plan during your pregnancy. Share your plan with your care provider. He may disagree with you about some things. You may prefer some things that the birth site won't allow. Discuss these things. Then change your birth site or birth plan as needed.

Maybe you and your prenatal care provider cannot agree. In that case, your provider should refer you to another prenatal care provider who shares your beliefs. This should not cost you more money. Prenatal care providers refer pregnant women to each other for many reasons.

## Birth Plan

| | |
|---|---|
| **Coaches** | I want to have my husband Jack and my sister Maria in the birthing room with me. |
| **Birthing position** | I plan to give birth in the squatting position or sitting up. I do not want to be lying down with my feet up. |
| **Medical steps** | I want to be able to walk around during labor. I prefer not to have a fetal monitor all the time.<br>I do not want to have an enema or be shaved.<br>I agree to have an episiotomy only if needed.<br>If the doctor suggests a C-section, I want to make the decision with her. |
| **Medication** | As long as the birth is going normally, I will decide if and when to have pain medication. |
| **After the birth** | My husband does not want to cut the umbilical cord.<br>If the baby is a boy, we want him circumcised.<br>I plan to breast-feed. If there are problems with feeding, I want to see a breast-feeding counselor. |

When you go to the hospital or birthing center to give birth, share your birth plan with the nurses and other care providers there.

---

Many labors don't happen just the way the mother and care providers want them to. You should be ready to change your birth plan as labor goes along. But a written plan gives you something to aim for.

## Breast-Feeding or Bottle-Feeding?

As part of your birth plan, you should decide whether you want to breast-feed or bottle-feed your baby. Whichever way you choose, you need to prepare ahead of time.

### Breast-feeding

- Your baby will get better nutrition from breast-feeding. Breast milk is the perfect food for babies. No artificial baby milk (formula) has the same benefits.
- Babies digest breast milk more easily than they digest formula.
- Babies who are breast-fed are less likely to be overweight.
- Breast-fed babies usually have fewer illnesses during the first year of life. They also have less chance of later diabetes.

- Babies' brains and language skills may develop better with breast milk.
- Breast-feeding is a special way to bond with your baby. It is joyful for many mothers.
- Breast milk costs nothing and is always there.
- Breast-feeding helps your uterus shrink back to its original size more quickly. It reduces the chances of breast or uterine cancer later in life.

If you plan to breast-feed, try to learn as much as possible about it before the baby is born. Talk to women who have breast-fed. Most communities have breast-feeding classes and consultants. Or you can get materials by calling the La Leche League: (800) LA-LECHE. They may also be able to tell you about classes and support groups in your area.

If you plan to breast-feed, consider these questions about your birth site:

- Does the staff promote breast-feeding?
- Does the staff know how to help a new mother breast-feed?
- Does it teach about the benefits of breast-feeding?
- Does it help mothers start breast-feeding within a half-hour of birth?

- Does it give newborns no food or drink other than breast milk, except for a medical reason?
- Does it allow mothers and infants to stay together 24 hours a day?
- Does it encourage breast-feeding whenever the baby wants?
- Does it put mothers in touch with breast-feeding support groups when they leave the birth site?

## Bottle-feeding

Bottle-feeding can be artificial baby milk (formula) or pumped breast milk.

- Bottle-feeding gives the mother more freedom. She doesn't have to be the one to feed the baby each time.
- Bottle-feeding allows the father or partner to share in the feeding.
- You may not be comfortable with the body contact that breast-feeding requires.

If you are breast-feeding you can express (pump) milk ahead of time. This lets someone else feed the baby if you won't be there. Some breast-fed babies need practice before they will take a bottle.

Pumps range in price. WIC offices and health departments often lend pumps to new mothers.

If you choose artificial milk, you may feel guilty because you have heard that breast-feeding is best. Experts agree that breast-feeding is better. But many healthy babies have been fed artificial milk. Perhaps you were one of them.

If you plan to use bottles, you should buy bottles, nipples, and brushes for cleaning the bottles and nipples.

## Things the Baby Needs

During your pregnancy, you should start collecting equipment and clothes for the baby. There are ways to cut down on the costs. You can

- accept used items gratefully. Your baby won't know or care that he's sleeping in a used crib. And clothes for newborns are often outgrown before they get very used.

- go to yard sales and second-hand stores. You can often pick up used clothing and equipment very cheaply. Check equipment carefully. Make sure its parts are all there and working. Check that it meets current safety standards.

- make a list of things you really need, in case people want gift ideas.
- find out about lending programs for infant car seats. They are often sponsored by hospitals, counties, and cities.

## What you really need

New equipment for babies comes out all the time. But babies don't really need very much.

Your baby will really need the following things:

**Crib.** Make sure the slats are no more than $2\,^3/_8$ inches apart and that none are damaged. Otherwise the baby could get her head caught between the slats. Use the guide below to check the slats on cribs you look at.

The mattress should fit snugly. If you can get more than two fingers between the edge of the mattress and the side of the crib, it's too loose.

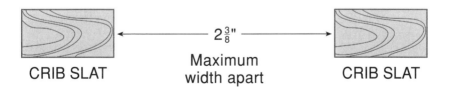

CRIB SLAT ← $2\frac{3}{8}$" → CRIB SLAT

Maximum width apart

Make sure the crib has no cutouts in the headboards and footboards that the baby could get her head stuck in. Make sure any latches are secure and couldn't be released easily by an older baby.

**Diapers.** You'll have to decide whether to use cloth or disposable diapers.

- Disposables are easier. Day care centers may require them. But they may cost more than cloth diapers (whether you use a diaper service or wash them yourself).
- Many people feel disposables are bad for the environment.
- Using cloth diapers can take a lot of effort. Cloth diapers sometimes have to be changed more often. If you wash them yourself, you may have to do it several times a week. On the other hand, washing your own diapers can save money.

**Clothes.** Babies, especially newborns, often need their clothes changed a couple of times each day. Think about how often you plan to do laundry. Get enough clothes to cover that number of days. Then get a few extra of everything.

Make sure all the clothes are washable, and buy them big. Your baby won't fit into newborn clothes for long.

**Blankets, sheets, and towels.** The thin blankets called receiving blankets have many uses. You can use them as burp cloths, to wrap the baby in, or to lay on the floor when you want to put him down.

You'll also need crib sheets and blankets.

**An infant car seat.** There are two types of car seats for infants:

- infant only
- infant/toddler convertible seats

When you are looking for a car seat, make sure that it

- has a label on it that says it meets Federal Motor Vehicle Safety Standard (FMVSS) 213
- has not been in an accident. If the person selling it doesn't know, don't buy it.
- has not been recalled for safety problems. Call (800) 424-9393 to find out.

A baby that weighs less than 20 pounds should be in the back seat in a rear-facing seat.

| Item | How many? |
| --- | --- |
| **diapers** | |
| cloth diapers | up to 100 if you wash weekly; 15 if you wash daily |
| diaper covers | 5 – 10 |
| disposable diapers | 80 – 100 a week |
| **clothes** | |
| undershirts | 4 – 6 |
| rompers (one-piece outfits) | 3 – 6 |
| sleepers | 2 – 4 |
| booties and socks | a few pairs |
| sweaters | 1 or 2 |
| hat | 1 |
| snowsuit | 1 in cold climates |
| **the crib** | |
| blankets | 4 – 6 |
| rubber sheets | 2 |
| fitted sheets | 2 – 4 |
| quilt | 1 |
| **for bathing** | |
| towels | 2 – 4 |
| washcloths | 4 – 8 |
| **big items** | |
| infant car seat | 1 |
| high chair | 1 |
| crib | 1 |
| **for feeding** | |
| nursing bras* | 2 |
| breast milk freezer storage bags* | a supply |
| breast pump* | 1 |
| bottles and nipples | 6 – 10 |
| bottle brush | 1 |
| nipple brush | 1 |
| **nice to have** | |
| stroller | 1 |
| baby backpack or carrier | 1 |
| playpen | 1 |
| changing table | 1 |
| diaper bag | 1 or 2 |

*You need these only if you're breast-feeding.

## Chapter 9

# Won't It Ever Be Over?

By your ninth month, it may seem as if you've been pregnant forever. You may feel big and awkward. You may have lots of little aches and pains. Nothing except the birth will make you smaller. But there are ways to feel more comfortable. Here are some symptoms and ways to ease them:

**Heartburn**

- Eat smaller, more frequent meals. Chew food well. Avoid greasy and spicy foods.
- Don't eat right before bedtime. If heartburn is worse when you're lying down, put several pillows under your head and back.
- Ask your doctor to suggest a safe antacid.

**Constipation** (difficulty moving your bowels)

- Exercise regularly.
- Eat high-fiber foods.
- Drink eight glasses of water a day.

**Varicose veins** (swollen and painful leg veins)

- Wear maternity support hose.
- Exercise regularly.
- If you sit for long periods of time, change position frequently and keep your feet up.
- Avoid crossing your legs.
- If you stand for long periods of time, rotate your feet at the ankle. Get off your feet for 15 minutes every 2 hours.

**Hemorrhoids** (swollen and painful veins near your anus)

- Avoid constipation.
- Sit on soft pillows.
- Soak in a warm bath.
- Apply ice packs.
- Ask your prenatal care provider to suggest a safe treatment.

**Backaches**

- Stand straight with your shoulders back.
- Wear low-heeled shoes.
- Don't lie flat on your back.
- When lifting, bend from the knees.

### Shortness of breath

- Do this deep-breathing exercise. Stand with your arms at your sides. Inhale slowly while you raise your arms as high as you can. Exhale slowly while you lower your arms. Repeat three to five times.

### Loss of bladder control

- Wear cotton panties and/or a panty shield.
- Do Kegel exercises.

  You can do Kegels lying on your back. But after your fourth month of pregnancy, you should do them sitting or standing.

  1. Tense the muscles around your vagina and anus, as when you stop your flow of urine.
  2. Hold as long as you can. Try to work up to holding for 10 seconds.
  3. Slowly relax your muscles.
  4. Repeat this up to 25 times a day.

### Leg cramps

- Flex your foot to stretch muscles.
- Use a heating pad.
- Soak in warm water.

### Hip pain

- Elevate your hips.
- Use heat and massage.

# Chapter 10

# Labor and Birth

When 40 weeks or so have passed, your baby is ready to be born. You may feel nervous. Learning about labor and delivery is one way to ease your concerns.

## Stages of Childbirth

There are three stages of childbirth:

1. **Labor.** In this first stage, contractions begin. Contractions are the tightening of the muscles of your womb (uterus). The contractions open up the mouth (cervix) of your womb.

| Stage | What's happening | Contractions | What you do |
|---|---|---|---|
| **Stage one — labor** | The cervix (opening of the womb) is opening. By the end of labor, it is open to 10 centimeters. | Mild at first; last about 60–90 seconds; happen every 15–20 minutes. Become stronger; last about 45 seconds, happen every 3 minutes. At the end of this stage, last about 60 seconds; happen every 2–3 minutes. Stage may last many hours. | Use the relaxation, breathing, and comfort exercises learned in childbirth classes. Your birthing care provider will probably tell you not to push. |
| **Stage two — birth** | The baby is ready to be pushed out. The baby is born. In a normal birth, the head slips out first. The body slips out with the next contractions. | Last about 60–90 seconds; happen every 2–5 minutes. | Push during contractions. Practice breathing and comfort exercises in between. |
| **Stage three — placenta delivery** | The placenta is pushed out after it detaches from the wall of the womb. | Less painful and closer together. This stage can take from 10 to 45 minutes. | Usually no pushing is needed. |

> If this is your first pregnancy, labor will probably last between 8 and 14 hours. If you have had a baby before, labor will probably be shorter.

2. **Birth.** This second stage usually lasts an hour or two. It can take even less time.
3. **Delivery of the placenta.** In this third stage, you push out the organ that has fed the baby while it grew in your body.

## How Do You Know You're in Labor?

Before their first child is born, many women worry that they won't know when labor has begun. In fact, it's very rare for a woman *not* to realize that she is in labor.

By the time you're ready to give birth, your body is usually giving you strong signals. If you're in labor, your contractions will

- get stronger and longer over time.
- probably start to come at regular intervals. The intervals will get shorter over time.
- begin in the lower back and spread to the lower stomach.
- get stronger even if you move around.

If you're not in labor, the contractions will

- stay irregular
- not get stronger
- start in the lower stomach, not the back
- go away if you move around

## When to Call Your Care Provider

When you call your birthing care provider, she will tell you when to leave for the birth site. The time depends on how far apart your contractions are coming. Most care providers will tell you to stay home until the contractions are coming every five minutes. When you can no longer walk or talk through a contraction, it is time to go to your birth site.

If your water breaks, some care providers will tell you to go to the birth site right away. Others will want to examine you first.

You may go into labor at night or on a weekend. Don't put off calling your care provider because of the time. People who deliver babies for a living are used to getting calls at all hours.

If you think it's time to go to the birth site, call your care provider, even if you're not sure.

## Arriving at the Birth Site

If you have preregistered at your birth site, the admitting process will be quicker. You may be able to go directly to the labor and birthing area. The staff at the birth site will probably ask you some questions. This is a good time to give them a copy of your birth plan.

After you are admitted, the staff will check

- your blood pressure
- your pulse
- your breathing
- your temperature

Someone will feel your belly to find out the position of the baby. A birthing care provider may do a vaginal exam also. This will tell them how far along your labor is.

In the past, most hospitals did certain things to prepare women for birth. These things included

- giving an enema
- putting in an IV drip
- shaving the pubic area
- not allowing the woman to eat
- making the woman stay in bed

These things are not usually necessary. As part of your birth plan, find out whether your birth site does any of them as a routine step.

## What to Bring to the Birth Site

A few weeks before your due date, you should pack a bag to bring to the birth site. It should include

- copies of your birth plan
- nightgowns
- a robe and slippers
- socks
- a nursing bra if you plan to breast-feed; a bra with firm support if you don't
- a brush, comb, toothbrush, toothpaste, soap, and shampoo
- phone numbers of friends and relatives
- clothes to take the baby home in
- comfortable clothes for your trip home (Your belly will still be larger than normal.)

Your childbirth teacher may suggest other items to bring with you.

## Positions for Labor

After your cervix opens to 10 centimeters, you will be ready to give birth.

Some positions can help labor progress. Others can slow it down. In general, you want to

- stay upright. This helps the contractions to work better. It also puts the baby's head at a better angle for birth. Contractions may be less painful if you are standing up.
- walk around as much as possible. This helps to keep you relaxed. It also can speed up labor.

If you have back pain, you may want to try the knee-chest position. It can ease the pain.

In later labor, you may need to lie down. Try not to lie flat on your back. This makes your body work harder. It can also cut down on the supply of oxygen to the baby.

## Positions for Birth

At the end of labor, the cervix is dilated to 10 centimeters. You may feel the urge to push. It's time to bring that baby into the world.

Certain positions are better for pushing.

# Positions for Labor

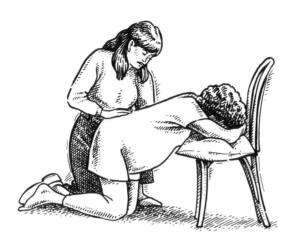

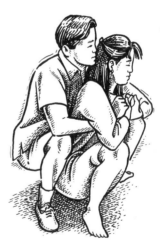

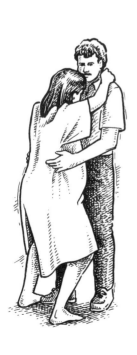

**Squatting.** At some birth sites, you can hang onto a bar for support when squatting. You can also hang onto your coach or the back of a chair.

Squatting may speed up the birth. Gravity will be working for you. Squatting also widens the opening of your pelvis. (With some medications, you will not be strong enough to squat.)

**Kneeling or sitting.** These positions also use gravity to speed up the birth.

**Side-lying.** This position makes it easy to rest between contractions.

## Procedures during Delivery

Sometimes your care provider will want to perform a procedure to help the delivery along. Many of these procedures are routine during births. If you don't want certain procedures used, say so in your birth plan. Of course, they may be needed if you have a special situation. Routine procedures include the following:

**Episiotomy.** An episiotomy is a cut made to enlarge the opening for the baby's head. It is done right before delivery. Some care providers do an episiotomy during every delivery. Others hardly use them at all.

Care providers who support episiotomies say they are easier to stitch up than the ragged tears that could happen otherwise. Those who oppose episiotomies say they are often larger than the tears that might happen naturally. They see no need for this as a routine step.

**Forceps delivery.** Forceps are a kind of tongs. Low forceps are sometimes used to pull the baby out when it seems to be stuck in the birth canal.

These days a cesarean birth is usually done instead of using high forceps. Cesarean births are described on pages 87 and 88.

**Suction delivery.** A vacuum extractor is sometimes used to pull the baby out of the birth canal when labor is stalled. It is not often used in the U.S.

## Medication during Labor and Birth

You may plan to get through labor and birth with no or little pain medication. The relaxation and comfort methods that are taught in childbirth classes should help with this. Check that the staff at your birth site knows about non-drug methods of pain relief.

If you want medication as part of the birth, you should know what the different medications are. You should also know their effects on mother, baby, and breast-feeding. This will help you choose wisely when the birth site staff asks if you want medication.

You'll get the best information on medications from your childbirth class or prenatal care provider. Ask what your options are and discuss them. Make sure your coach knows what you have decided.

## Induced Labor

Sometimes your care provider may want to make labor start. This is called inducing labor. Your care provider may want to do this if

- you are at least two weeks past your due date
- the baby isn't well
- your water has broken, but labor hasn't started
- you have an illness that threatens you or your baby
- your labor is weak or has stopped

If your care provider wants to induce labor, ask why. If it's because your health or the baby's health is at risk, it may be the best choice.

But if it seems that your care provider wants to induce labor for his or her convenience, you should question it. Labor can't be induced unless you give permission. If you do give permission for labor to be induced, you will get medication. Labor will probably start about 30 minutes later.

Inducing labor will cause contractions to start suddenly and strongly. Because of this, your relaxation and comfort measures may not work as well. You may want pain medication. Induced labors also lead to cesarean births more often.

If labor doesn't start after six to eight hours, the next step may be a cesarean birth.

## Cesarean Births (C-Sections)

In some cases, the baby can't be born through the vagina. Surgery called a cesarean birth (or C-section) is performed. When a woman has a cesarean birth, her baby is pulled out through a cut in the wall of the uterus.

The reasons for having a cesarean birth fall into three groups:

**Problems with the baby.** The surgery is often performed because the baby is at risk, such as not getting enough oxygen.

The surgery may be done if the baby is in a breech position (coming feet or buttocks first). The baby is lying the wrong way for birth. In some cases, this can be avoided. Exercises can sometimes turn the baby around. Sometimes the doctor or nurse-midwife helps turn the baby. Cesarean births are no longer done routinely for breech births.

**Problems with the birth passage.** Sometimes the baby's head is too large to pass through the bones of the mother's pelvis.

**Failure to progress.** Sometimes the mother labors for hours and hours, but the cervix doesn't open as much as it needs to.

Many experts say too many babies are born by cesarean birth. They say some doctors perform the surgery because they are impatient with long labors. Doctors may tell women who have one cesarean birth that any later babies must also be born that way. This is not true. About 70 percent of women succeed if they try VBAC (vaginal birth after cesarean).

If you have had a cesarean birth and want to try VBAC, talk to your birthing care provider. Find out if he will support you in trying a VBAC. If not, and if there is no clear reason, you may need to find another care provider.

# Chapter 11

# After the Birth

The first few weeks after you give birth are called the postpartum period. You have been looking forward to this time for months. But you may not feel the way you thought you would. You may feel

- very tired.
- very happy or depressed (the blues). You may also swing between the two moods.
- afraid.

Your body probably doesn't feel great yet either.

☞ ▬ ▬ ▬ ▬ ▬ ▬ ▬ ▬ ▬ ▬ ▬ ▬ ▬ ▬ ▬ ▬ ▬ ▬ ▬ ▬ ▬ ▬ ┐
Giving birth may be the biggest change your body
ever experiences. It takes time to recover.

The best thing to do right after giving birth is to take it easy and rest. Give yourself time to recover and adjust to your new role.

In many parts of the world, new mothers are waited on for a month or so after giving birth. Ask your friends and family to help you. In most cases, they'll be thrilled to help out.

## Bonding

You may feel love for your child from the very first moment. Or you may not. After all, you're likely to be worn out when you get your first look at her. And even though you've carried this baby in your body for months, it will take time to get to know her.

Some mothers worry if they don't feel a rush of love right away. They fear they will never bond with their child. But bonding doesn't have to happen in an instant. The feelings build up over months and years of caring for a child.

## Starting to Breast-Feed

It may seem that breast-feeding should be the most natural thing in the world. But both mother and baby sometimes need to learn how to do it.

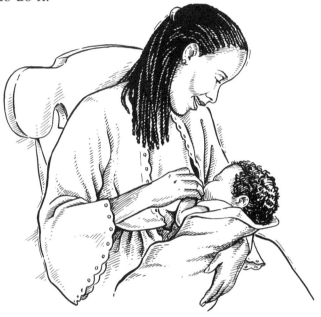

Keep your baby with you after birth if you can. That way, you can let him breast-feed as soon as he starts mouthing and looking for the nipple. Babies who are able to breast-feed within the first hour or so after birth usually breast-feed well.

Some babies take several days to learn to breast-feed. This is sometimes true if you had pain medication during delivery. Be patient and give the baby lots of time to rest and nuzzle near your nipple. Ask for a lactation consultant (breast-feeding counselor) to help if needed.

At first, you may notice that even when the baby sucks on your breast, not much comes out. That's OK. It takes a few days for your milk to come in quantity. The more minutes the baby spends at the breast the sooner that happens.

At first the baby will get colostrum. That is a thick yellow early milk. Colostrum gives the newborn baby some protection from disease.

When your milk comes in, your breasts may swell. This is called engorgement. Frequent feedings prevent engorgement. Applying cold packs can help reduce it.

At first, your nipples may also be sore from the baby sucking on them. Proper positioning of the baby at the breast reduces nipple soreness. The soreness will go away in time.

You may feel more confident about breast-feeding if you speak to a lactation consultant. If you gave birth in a hospital or birthing center, there is probably one on staff. If not, ask your care provider how to get in touch with one.

## Circumcision

If you have a boy, you will have to decide whether to have him circumcised. Circumcision is the removal of part of the foreskin of the baby's penis. If done, this procedure is usually performed in the first day or two after birth. It's sometimes later if it is part of a religious ceremony.

Among Jews and Muslims, circumcision is done for religious reasons. In the U.S., many other parents have their sons circumcised too.

There is a lot of debate over whether boys should be circumcised. A few years ago, the American Academy of Pediatrics advised against it. Now it says parents, along with the baby's doctor, should make the decision.

## Conclusion

Remember that you have lots of support. Lean on your family, friends, and community members to help you. Or find local support groups for special advice or help. Call your local department of social services or health for help if you are having trouble paying to feed and take care of your child.

Ask questions at every stage. Use all the help you can get. Most of all, enjoy and be proud of your child.

# Philosophy of Birth, ASPO/Lamaze

**B**irth is normal, natural, and healthy.

**T**he experience of birth profoundly affects women and their families.

**W**omen's inner wisdom guides them through birth.

**W**omen's confidence and ability to give birth is either enhanced or diminished by the care provider and place of birth.

**W**omen have a right to give birth free from routine medical interventions.

**B**irth can safely take place in birth centers and homes.

**C**hildbirth education empowers women to make informed choices in health care, to assume responsibility for their health, and to trust their inner wisdom.

# Resources

You can find more information on pregnancy and childbirth. Try these places.

## Books and videos for the next stage

Your local library or bookstore probably has many books and videos about raising children. Signal Hill Publications publishes a quick and easy guide called *The Safe, Self-Confident Child.* You should be able to get that book at the same place you got this one. Or call (800) 506-READ to order it.

## Breast-Feeding

La Leche League International, Inc.
(800) LA-LECHE

## Childbirth Education

American Society for Psychoprophylaxis in Obstetrics (ASPO/Lamaze)
(800) 368-4404

American Academy of Husband-Coached Childbirth (The Bradley Method Pregnancy Hotline)
(800) 423-2397

International Childbirth Education Association (ICEA)
(612) 854-8660

International Association of Parents and Professionals
for Safe Alternatives in Childbirth (NAPSAC)
> (573) 238-2010

## Cesarean Births

Cesareans/Support, Education and Concern (C/SEC)
> (508) 877-8266

International Cesarean Awareness Network (ICAN)
> (315) 424-1942

## Home Birth

Informed Homebirth, Inc.·
> (313) 662-6857

## Safety of Baby Equipment

U.S. Consumer Product Safety Commission
> (800) 638-2772

## High-Risk Pregnancies

Sidelines National Support Network
> (714) 497-2265

## Nutrition

Special Supplemental Food for Women, Infants and
Children (WIC)
> Call your local department of social services.

Children's Foundation
> (202) 347-3300